EAT THIS, NOT THAT DIET
TRACK YOUR WEIGHT LOSS PROGRESS
WITH BMI CHART

Copyright 2015

WEIGHT CATEGORIES

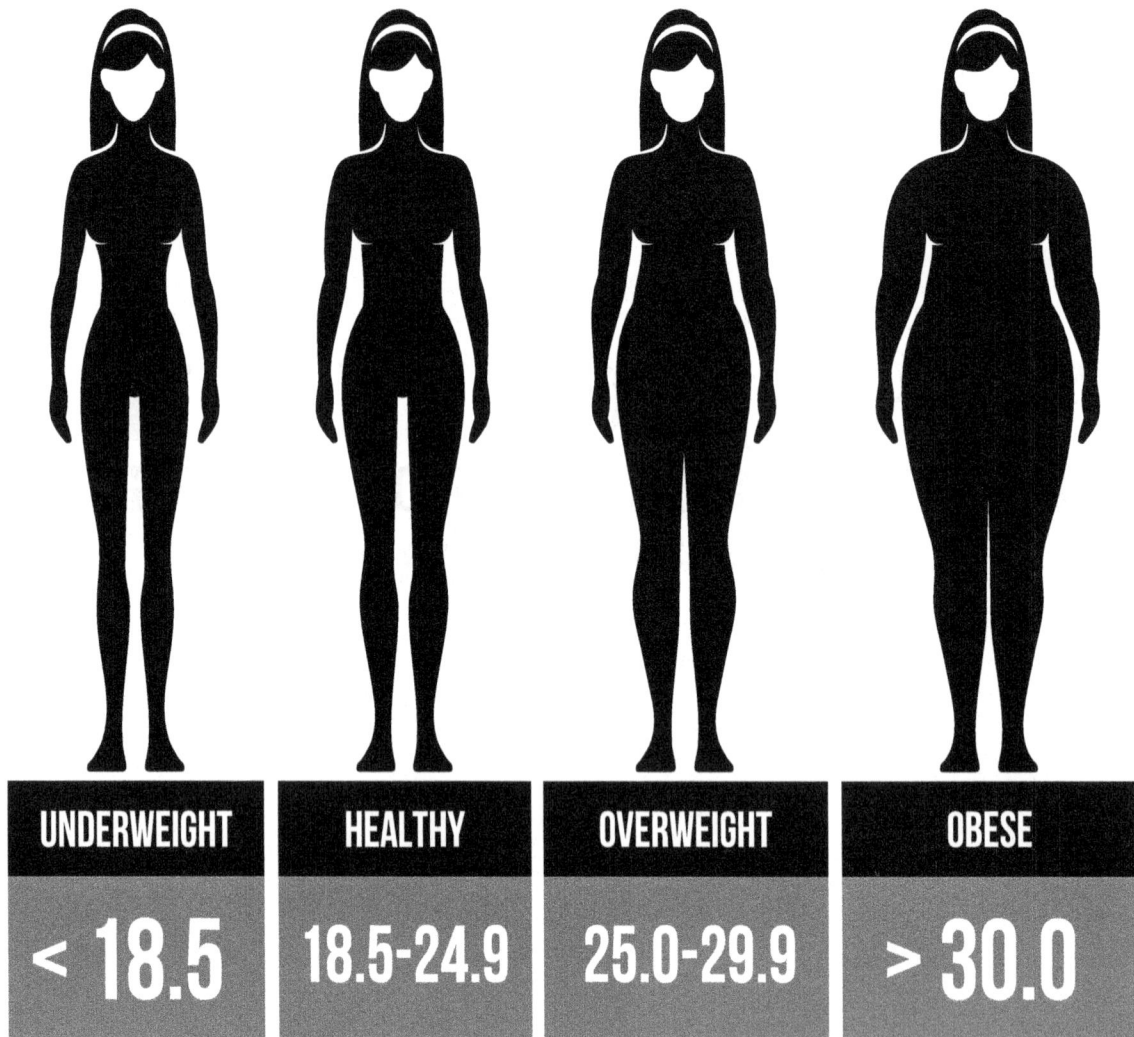

UNDERWEIGHT	HEALTHY	OVERWEIGHT	OBESE
< 18.5	18.5-24.9	25.0-29.9	> 30.0

MY DAILY PLAN

_____

_____

_____

_____

Before Pictures Here

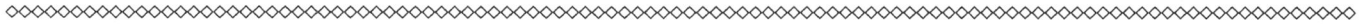

◇◇

After Pictures Here

DIET JOURNAL

Date: _____

FOOD and BEVERAGE	CALORIE	FIBER	PROTEIN	CARB	FAT
BREAKFAST					
Breakfast Total >					
LUNCH					
Lunch Total >					
DINNER					
Dinner Total >					

SPECIAL DIETARY NOTES:

DIET JOURNAL

Date: _____

FOOD and BEVERAGE	CALORIE	FIBER	PROTEIN	CARB	FAT
BREAKFAST					
Breakfast Total >					
LUNCH					
Lunch Total >					
DINNER					
Dinner Total >					

SPECIAL DIETARY NOTES:

_____
_____
_____
_____
_____
_____
_____
_____
_____
_____
_____
_____
_____
_____
_____
_____

DIET JOURNAL

Date: _____

FOOD and BEVERAGE	CALORIE	FIBER	PROTEIN	CARB	FAT
BREAKFAST					
Breakfast Total >					
LUNCH					
Lunch Total >					
DINNER					
Dinner Total >					

SPECIAL DIETARY NOTES:

_____
_____
_____
_____
_____
_____
_____
_____
_____
_____
_____
_____
_____
_____
_____

DIET JOURNAL

Date: _____

FOOD and BEVERAGE	CALORIE	FIBER	PROTEIN	CARB	FAT
BREAKFAST					
Breakfast Total >					
LUNCH					
Lunch Total >					
DINNER					
Dinner Total >					

SPECIAL DIETARY NOTES:

_____
_____
_____
_____
_____
_____
_____
_____
_____
_____
_____
_____
_____
_____
_____

DIET JOURNAL

Date: _____

FOOD and BEVERAGE	CALORIE	FIBER	PROTEIN	CARB	FAT
BREAKFAST					
Breakfast Total >					
LUNCH					
Lunch Total >					
DINNER					
Dinner Total >					

SPECIAL DIETARY NOTES:

DIET JOURNAL

Date: _____

FOOD and BEVERAGE	CALORIE	FIBER	PROTEIN	CARB	FAT
BREAKFAST					
Breakfast Total >					
LUNCH					
Lunch Total >					
DINNER					
Dinner Total >					

SPECIAL DIETARY NOTES:

_____
_____
_____
_____
_____
_____
_____
_____
_____
_____
_____
_____
_____
_____
_____
_____
_____

DIET JOURNAL

Date: _____

FOOD and BEVERAGE	CALORIE	FIBER	PROTEIN	CARB	FAT
BREAKFAST					
Breakfast Total >					
LUNCH					
Lunch Total >					
DINNER					
Dinner Total >					

SPECIAL DIETARY NOTES:

_____
_____
_____
_____
_____
_____
_____
_____
_____
_____
_____
_____
_____
_____
_____
_____

DIET JOURNAL

Date: _____

FOOD and BEVERAGE	CALORIE	FIBER	PROTEIN	CARB	FAT
BREAKFAST					
Breakfast Total >					
LUNCH					
Lunch Total >					
DINNER					
Dinner Total >					

SPECIAL DIETARY NOTES:

DIET JOURNAL

Date: _____

FOOD and BEVERAGE	CALORIE	FIBER	PROTEIN	CARB	FAT
BREAKFAST					
Breakfast Total >					
LUNCH					
Lunch Total >					
DINNER					
Dinner Total >					

SPECIAL DIETARY NOTES:

_____
_____
_____
_____
_____
_____
_____
_____
_____
_____
_____
_____
_____
_____
_____
_____

DIET JOURNAL

Date: _____

FOOD and BEVERAGE	CALORIE	FIBER	PROTEIN	CARB	FAT
BREAKFAST					
Breakfast Total >					
LUNCH					
Lunch Total >					
DINNER					
Dinner Total >					

SPECIAL DIETARY NOTES:

DIET JOURNAL

Date: _____

FOOD and BEVERAGE	CALORIE	FIBER	PROTEIN	CARB	FAT
BREAKFAST					
Breakfast Total >					
LUNCH					
Lunch Total >					
DINNER					
Dinner Total >					

SPECIAL DIETARY NOTES:

_____
_____
_____
_____
_____
_____
_____
_____
_____
_____
_____
_____
_____
_____
_____
_____

DIET JOURNAL

Date: _____

FOOD and BEVERAGE	CALORIE	FIBER	PROTEIN	CARB	FAT
BREAKFAST					
Breakfast Total >					
LUNCH					
Lunch Total >					
DINNER					
Dinner Total >					

SPECIAL DIETARY NOTES:

_____
_____
_____
_____
_____
_____
_____
_____
_____
_____
_____
_____
_____
_____
_____
_____

DIET JOURNAL

Date: _____

FOOD and BEVERAGE	CALORIE	FIBER	PROTEIN	CARB	FAT
BREAKFAST					
Breakfast Total >					
LUNCH					
Lunch Total >					
DINNER					
Dinner Total >					

SPECIAL DIETARY NOTES:

_____
_____
_____
_____
_____
_____
_____
_____
_____
_____
_____
_____
_____
_____
_____
_____

DIET JOURNAL

Date: _____

FOOD and BEVERAGE	CALORIE	FIBER	PROTEIN	CARB	FAT
BREAKFAST					
Breakfast Total >					
LUNCH					
Lunch Total >					
DINNER					
Dinner Total >					

SPECIAL DIETARY NOTES:

_____
_____
_____
_____
_____
_____
_____
_____
_____
_____
_____
_____
_____
_____
_____

DIET JOURNAL

Date: _____

FOOD and BEVERAGE	CALORIE	FIBER	PROTEIN	CARB	FAT
BREAKFAST					
Breakfast Total >					
LUNCH					
Lunch Total >					
DINNER					
Dinner Total >					

SPECIAL DIETARY NOTES:

_____
_____
_____
_____
_____
_____
_____
_____
_____
_____
_____
_____
_____
_____
_____
_____
_____

DIET JOURNAL

Date: _____

FOOD and BEVERAGE	CALORIE	FIBER	PROTEIN	CARB	FAT
BREAKFAST					
Breakfast Total >					
LUNCH					
Lunch Total >					
DINNER					
Dinner Total >					

SPECIAL DIETARY NOTES:

_____
_____
_____
_____
_____
_____
_____
_____
_____
_____
_____
_____
_____
_____
_____
_____

DIET JOURNAL

Date: _____

FOOD and BEVERAGE	CALORIE	FIBER	PROTEIN	CARB	FAT
BREAKFAST					
Breakfast Total >					
LUNCH					
Lunch Total >					
DINNER					
Dinner Total >					

SPECIAL DIETARY NOTES:

_____
_____
_____
_____
_____
_____
_____
_____
_____
_____
_____
_____
_____
_____
_____
_____
_____
_____

DIET JOURNAL

Date: _____

FOOD and BEVERAGE	CALORIE	FIBER	PROTEIN	CARB	FAT
BREAKFAST					
Breakfast Total >					
LUNCH					
Lunch Total >					
DINNER					
Dinner Total >					

SPECIAL DIETARY NOTES:

_____
_____
_____
_____
_____
_____
_____
_____
_____
_____
_____
_____
_____
_____
_____
_____

DIET JOURNAL

Date: _____

FOOD and BEVERAGE	CALORIE	FIBER	PROTEIN	CARB	FAT
BREAKFAST					
Breakfast Total >					
LUNCH					
Lunch Total >					
DINNER					
Dinner Total >					

SPECIAL DIETARY NOTES:

_____
_____
_____
_____
_____
_____
_____
_____
_____
_____
_____
_____
_____
_____
_____
_____

DIET JOURNAL

Date: _____

FOOD and BEVERAGE	CALORIE	FIBER	PROTEIN	CARB	FAT
BREAKFAST					
Breakfast Total >					
LUNCH					
Lunch Total >					
DINNER					
Dinner Total >					

SPECIAL DIETARY NOTES:

_____
_____
_____
_____
_____
_____
_____
_____
_____
_____
_____
_____
_____
_____
_____

DIET JOURNAL

Date: _____

FOOD and BEVERAGE	CALORIE	FIBER	PROTEIN	CARB	FAT
BREAKFAST					
Breakfast Total >					
LUNCH					
Lunch Total >					
DINNER					
Dinner Total >					

SPECIAL DIETARY NOTES:

_____
_____
_____
_____
_____
_____
_____
_____
_____
_____
_____
_____
_____
_____
_____

DIET JOURNAL

Date: _____

FOOD and BEVERAGE	CALORIE	FIBER	PROTEIN	CARB	FAT
BREAKFAST					
Breakfast Total >					
LUNCH					
Lunch Total >					
DINNER					
Dinner Total >					

SPECIAL DIETARY NOTES:

_____
_____
_____
_____
_____
_____
_____
_____
_____
_____
_____
_____
_____
_____
_____

DIET JOURNAL

Date: _____

FOOD and BEVERAGE	CALORIE	FIBER	PROTEIN	CARB	FAT
BREAKFAST					
Breakfast Total >					
LUNCH					
Lunch Total >					
DINNER					
Dinner Total >					

SPECIAL DIETARY NOTES:

_____
_____
_____
_____
_____
_____
_____
_____
_____
_____
_____
_____
_____
_____
_____

DIET JOURNAL

Date: _____

FOOD and BEVERAGE	CALORIE	FIBER	PROTEIN	CARB	FAT
BREAKFAST					
Breakfast Total >					
LUNCH					
Lunch Total >					
DINNER					
Dinner Total >					

SPECIAL DIETARY NOTES:

_____
_____
_____
_____
_____
_____
_____
_____
_____
_____
_____
_____
_____
_____
_____

DIET JOURNAL

Date: _____

FOOD and BEVERAGE	CALORIE	FIBER	PROTEIN	CARB	FAT
BREAKFAST					
Breakfast Total >					
LUNCH					
Lunch Total >					
DINNER					
Dinner Total >					

SPECIAL DIETARY NOTES:

_____
_____
_____
_____
_____
_____
_____
_____
_____
_____
_____
_____
_____
_____
_____
_____
_____

DIET JOURNAL

Date: _____

FOOD and BEVERAGE	CALORIE	FIBER	PROTEIN	CARB	FAT
BREAKFAST					
Breakfast Total >					
LUNCH					
Lunch Total >					
DINNER					
Dinner Total >					

SPECIAL DIETARY NOTES:

_____
_____
_____
_____
_____
_____
_____
_____
_____
_____
_____
_____
_____
_____
_____
_____

DIET JOURNAL

Date: _____

FOOD and BEVERAGE	CALORIE	FIBER	PROTEIN	CARB	FAT
BREAKFAST					
Breakfast Total >					
LUNCH					
Lunch Total >					
DINNER					
Dinner Total >					

SPECIAL DIETARY NOTES:

_____

_____

_____

_____

_____

_____

_____

_____

_____

_____

_____

_____

_____

_____

_____

_____

DIET JOURNAL

Date: _____

FOOD and BEVERAGE	CALORIE	FIBER	PROTEIN	CARB	FAT
BREAKFAST					
Breakfast Total >					
LUNCH					
Lunch Total >					
DINNER					
Dinner Total >					

SPECIAL DIETARY NOTES:

_____
_____
_____
_____
_____
_____
_____
_____
_____
_____
_____
_____
_____
_____

DIET JOURNAL

Date: _____

FOOD and BEVERAGE	CALORIE	FIBER	PROTEIN	CARB	FAT
BREAKFAST					
Breakfast Total >					
LUNCH					
Lunch Total >					
DINNER					
Dinner Total >					

SPECIAL DIETARY NOTES:

_____
_____
_____
_____
_____
_____
_____
_____
_____
_____
_____
_____
_____
_____
_____

DIET JOURNAL

Date: _____

FOOD and BEVERAGE	CALORIE	FIBER	PROTEIN	CARB	FAT
BREAKFAST					
Breakfast Total >					
LUNCH					
Lunch Total >					
DINNER					
Dinner Total >					

SPECIAL DIETARY NOTES:

_____
_____
_____
_____
_____
_____
_____
_____
_____
_____
_____
_____
_____
_____
_____
_____
_____

DIET JOURNAL

Date: _____

FOOD and BEVERAGE	CALORIE	FIBER	PROTEIN	CARB	FAT
BREAKFAST					
Breakfast Total >					
LUNCH					
Lunch Total >					
DINNER					
Dinner Total >					

SPECIAL DIETARY NOTES:

_____
_____
_____
_____
_____
_____
_____
_____
_____
_____
_____
_____
_____
_____
_____

DIET JOURNAL

Date: _____

FOOD and BEVERAGE	CALORIE	FIBER	PROTEIN	CARB	FAT
BREAKFAST					
Breakfast Total >					
LUNCH					
Lunch Total >					
DINNER					
Dinner Total >					

SPECIAL DIETARY NOTES:

_____
_____
_____
_____
_____
_____
_____
_____
_____
_____
_____
_____
_____
_____
_____
_____

DIET JOURNAL

Date: _____

FOOD and BEVERAGE	CALORIE	FIBER	PROTEIN	CARB	FAT
BREAKFAST					
Breakfast Total >					
LUNCH					
Lunch Total >					
DINNER					
Dinner Total >					

SPECIAL DIETARY NOTES:

_____
_____
_____
_____
_____
_____
_____
_____
_____
_____
_____
_____
_____
_____
_____

DIET JOURNAL

Date: _____

FOOD and BEVERAGE	CALORIE	FIBER	PROTEIN	CARB	FAT
BREAKFAST					
Breakfast Total >					
LUNCH					
Lunch Total >					
DINNER					
Dinner Total >					

SPECIAL DIETARY NOTES:

_____
_____
_____
_____
_____
_____
_____
_____
_____
_____
_____
_____
_____
_____
_____
_____

DIET JOURNAL

Date: _____

FOOD and BEVERAGE	CALORIE	FIBER	PROTEIN	CARB	FAT
BREAKFAST					
Breakfast Total >					
LUNCH					
Lunch Total >					
DINNER					
Dinner Total >					

SPECIAL DIETARY NOTES:

_____
_____
_____
_____
_____
_____
_____
_____
_____
_____
_____
_____
_____
_____
_____
_____
_____

DIET JOURNAL

Date: _____

FOOD and BEVERAGE	CALORIE	FIBER	PROTEIN	CARB	FAT
BREAKFAST					
Breakfast Total >					
LUNCH					
Lunch Total >					
DINNER					
Dinner Total >					

SPECIAL DIETARY NOTES:

_____
_____
_____
_____
_____
_____
_____
_____
_____
_____
_____
_____
_____
_____
_____

DIET JOURNAL

Date: _____

FOOD and BEVERAGE	CALORIE	FIBER	PROTEIN	CARB	FAT
BREAKFAST					
Breakfast Total >					
LUNCH					
Lunch Total >					
DINNER					
Dinner Total >					

SPECIAL DIETARY NOTES:

_____
_____
_____
_____
_____
_____
_____
_____
_____
_____
_____
_____
_____
_____
_____
_____

DIET JOURNAL

Date: _____

FOOD and BEVERAGE	CALORIE	FIBER	PROTEIN	CARB	FAT
BREAKFAST					
Breakfast Total >					
LUNCH					
Lunch Total >					
DINNER					
Dinner Total >					

SPECIAL DIETARY NOTES:

_____
_____
_____
_____
_____
_____
_____
_____
_____
_____
_____
_____
_____
_____
_____

DIET JOURNAL

Date: _____

FOOD and BEVERAGE	CALORIE	FIBER	PROTEIN	CARB	FAT
BREAKFAST					
Breakfast Total >					
LUNCH					
Lunch Total >					
DINNER					
Dinner Total >					

SPECIAL DIETARY NOTES:

_____
_____
_____
_____
_____
_____
_____
_____
_____
_____
_____
_____
_____
_____
_____
_____
_____

DIET JOURNAL

Date: _____

FOOD and BEVERAGE	CALORIE	FIBER	PROTEIN	CARB	FAT
BREAKFAST					
Breakfast Total >					
LUNCH					
Lunch Total >					
DINNER					
Dinner Total >					

SPECIAL DIETARY NOTES:

_____
_____
_____
_____
_____
_____
_____
_____
_____
_____
_____
_____
_____
_____
_____

DIET JOURNAL

Date: _____

FOOD and BEVERAGE	CALORIE	FIBER	PROTEIN	CARB	FAT
BREAKFAST					
Breakfast Total >					
LUNCH					
Lunch Total >					
DINNER					
Dinner Total >					

SPECIAL DIETARY NOTES:

_____
_____
_____
_____
_____
_____
_____
_____
_____
_____
_____
_____
_____
_____
_____
_____

DIET JOURNAL

Date: _____

FOOD and BEVERAGE	CALORIE	FIBER	PROTEIN	CARB	FAT
BREAKFAST					
Breakfast Total >					
LUNCH					
Lunch Total >					
DINNER					
Dinner Total >					

SPECIAL DIETARY NOTES:

DIET JOURNAL

Date: _____

FOOD and BEVERAGE	CALORIE	FIBER	PROTEIN	CARB	FAT
BREAKFAST					
Breakfast Total >					
LUNCH					
Lunch Total >					
DINNER					
Dinner Total >					

SPECIAL DIETARY NOTES:

_____
_____
_____
_____
_____
_____
_____
_____
_____
_____
_____
_____
_____
_____
_____
_____

DIET JOURNAL

Date: _____

FOOD and BEVERAGE	CALORIE	FIBER	PROTEIN	CARB	FAT
BREAKFAST					
Breakfast Total >					
LUNCH					
Lunch Total >					
DINNER					
Dinner Total >					

SPECIAL DIETARY NOTES:

_____
_____
_____
_____
_____
_____
_____
_____
_____
_____
_____
_____
_____
_____
_____

DIET JOURNAL

Date: _____

FOOD and BEVERAGE	CALORIE	FIBER	PROTEIN	CARB	FAT
BREAKFAST					
Breakfast Total >					
LUNCH					
Lunch Total >					
DINNER					
Dinner Total >					

SPECIAL DIETARY NOTES:

_____
_____
_____
_____
_____
_____
_____
_____
_____
_____
_____
_____
_____
_____
_____
_____

DIET JOURNAL

Date: _____

FOOD and BEVERAGE	CALORIE	FIBER	PROTEIN	CARB	FAT
BREAKFAST					
Breakfast Total >					
LUNCH					
Lunch Total >					
DINNER					
Dinner Total >					

SPECIAL DIETARY NOTES:

_____
_____
_____
_____
_____
_____
_____
_____
_____
_____
_____
_____
_____
_____
_____
_____

DIET JOURNAL

Date: _____

FOOD and BEVERAGE	CALORIE	FIBER	PROTEIN	CARB	FAT
BREAKFAST					
Breakfast Total >					
LUNCH					
Lunch Total >					
DINNER					
Dinner Total >					

SPECIAL DIETARY NOTES:

_____
_____
_____
_____
_____
_____
_____
_____
_____
_____
_____
_____
_____
_____
_____
_____
_____
_____

DIET JOURNAL

Date: _____

FOOD and BEVERAGE	CALORIE	FIBER	PROTEIN	CARB	FAT
BREAKFAST					
Breakfast Total >					
LUNCH					
Lunch Total >					
DINNER					
Dinner Total >					

SPECIAL DIETARY NOTES:

DIET JOURNAL

Date: _____

FOOD and BEVERAGE	CALORIE	FIBER	PROTEIN	CARB	FAT
BREAKFAST					
Breakfast Total >					
LUNCH					
Lunch Total >					
DINNER					
Dinner Total >					

SPECIAL DIETARY NOTES:

_____
_____
_____
_____
_____
_____
_____
_____
_____
_____
_____
_____
_____
_____
_____
_____

DIET JOURNAL

Date: _____

FOOD and BEVERAGE	CALORIE	FIBER	PROTEIN	CARB	FAT
BREAKFAST					
Breakfast Total >					
LUNCH					
Lunch Total >					
DINNER					
Dinner Total >					

SPECIAL DIETARY NOTES:

_____
_____
_____
_____
_____
_____
_____
_____
_____
_____
_____
_____
_____
_____
_____
_____
_____

DIET JOURNAL

Date: _____

FOOD and BEVERAGE	CALORIE	FIBER	PROTEIN	CARB	FAT
BREAKFAST					
Breakfast Total >					
LUNCH					
Lunch Total >					
DINNER					
Dinner Total >					

SPECIAL DIETARY NOTES:

DIET JOURNAL

Date: _____

FOOD and BEVERAGE	CALORIE	FIBER	PROTEIN	CARB	FAT
BREAKFAST					
Breakfast Total >					
LUNCH					
Lunch Total >					
DINNER					
Dinner Total >					

SPECIAL DIETARY NOTES:

_____
_____
_____
_____
_____
_____
_____
_____
_____
_____
_____
_____
_____
_____

DIET JOURNAL

Date: _____

FOOD and BEVERAGE	CALORIE	FIBER	PROTEIN	CARB	FAT
BREAKFAST					
Breakfast Total >					
LUNCH					
Lunch Total >					
DINNER					
Dinner Total >					

SPECIAL DIETARY NOTES:

_____
_____
_____
_____
_____
_____
_____
_____
_____
_____
_____
_____
_____
_____
_____
_____

DIET JOURNAL

Date: _____

FOOD and BEVERAGE	CALORIE	FIBER	PROTEIN	CARB	FAT
BREAKFAST					
Breakfast Total >					
LUNCH					
Lunch Total >					
DINNER					
Dinner Total >					

SPECIAL DIETARY NOTES:

_____
_____
_____
_____
_____
_____
_____
_____
_____
_____
_____
_____
_____
_____
_____
_____

DIET JOURNAL

Date: _____

FOOD and BEVERAGE	CALORIE	FIBER	PROTEIN	CARB	FAT
BREAKFAST					
Breakfast Total >					
LUNCH					
Lunch Total >					
DINNER					
Dinner Total >					

SPECIAL DIETARY NOTES:

_____
_____
_____
_____
_____
_____
_____
_____
_____
_____
_____
_____
_____
_____

DIET JOURNAL

Date: _____

FOOD and BEVERAGE	CALORIE	FIBER	PROTEIN	CARB	FAT
BREAKFAST					
Breakfast Total >					
LUNCH					
Lunch Total >					
DINNER					
Dinner Total >					

SPECIAL DIETARY NOTES:

_____
_____
_____
_____
_____
_____
_____
_____
_____
_____
_____
_____
_____
_____
_____
_____
_____

DIET JOURNAL

Date: _____

FOOD and BEVERAGE	CALORIE	FIBER	PROTEIN	CARB	FAT
BREAKFAST					
Breakfast Total >					
LUNCH					
Lunch Total >					
DINNER					
Dinner Total >					

SPECIAL DIETARY NOTES:

_____
_____
_____
_____
_____
_____
_____
_____
_____
_____
_____
_____
_____
_____
_____

DIET JOURNAL

Date: _____

FOOD and BEVERAGE	CALORIE	FIBER	PROTEIN	CARB	FAT
BREAKFAST					
Breakfast Total >					
LUNCH					
Lunch Total >					
DINNER					
Dinner Total >					

SPECIAL DIETARY NOTES:

_____
_____
_____
_____
_____
_____
_____
_____
_____
_____
_____
_____
_____
_____
_____

DIET JOURNAL

Date: _____

FOOD and BEVERAGE	CALORIE	FIBER	PROTEIN	CARB	FAT
BREAKFAST					
Breakfast Total >					
LUNCH					
Lunch Total >					
DINNER					
Dinner Total >					

SPECIAL DIETARY NOTES:

_____
_____
_____
_____
_____
_____
_____
_____
_____
_____
_____
_____
_____
_____
_____
_____

DIET JOURNAL

Date: _____

FOOD and BEVERAGE	CALORIE	FIBER	PROTEIN	CARB	FAT
BREAKFAST					
Breakfast Total >					
LUNCH					
Lunch Total >					
DINNER					
Dinner Total >					

SPECIAL DIETARY NOTES:

_____
_____
_____
_____
_____
_____
_____
_____
_____
_____
_____
_____
_____
_____
_____
_____

DIET JOURNAL

Date: _____

FOOD and BEVERAGE	CALORIE	FIBER	PROTEIN	CARB	FAT
BREAKFAST					
Breakfast Total >					
LUNCH					
Lunch Total >					
DINNER					
Dinner Total >					

SPECIAL DIETARY NOTES:

_____
_____
_____
_____
_____
_____
_____
_____
_____
_____
_____
_____
_____
_____
_____

DIET JOURNAL

Date: _____

FOOD and BEVERAGE	CALORIE	FIBER	PROTEIN	CARB	FAT
BREAKFAST					
Breakfast Total >					
LUNCH					
Lunch Total >					
DINNER					
Dinner Total >					

SPECIAL DIETARY NOTES:

_____
_____
_____
_____
_____
_____
_____
_____
_____
_____
_____
_____
_____
_____
_____
_____

DIET JOURNAL

Date: _____

FOOD and BEVERAGE	CALORIE	FIBER	PROTEIN	CARB	FAT
BREAKFAST					
Breakfast Total >					
LUNCH					
Lunch Total >					
DINNER					
Dinner Total >					

SPECIAL DIETARY NOTES:

_____
_____
_____
_____
_____
_____
_____
_____
_____
_____
_____
_____
_____
_____
_____
_____

DIET JOURNAL

Date: _____

FOOD and BEVERAGE	CALORIE	FIBER	PROTEIN	CARB	FAT
BREAKFAST					
Breakfast Total >					
LUNCH					
Lunch Total >					
DINNER					
Dinner Total >					

SPECIAL DIETARY NOTES:

_____
_____
_____
_____
_____
_____
_____
_____
_____
_____
_____
_____
_____
_____
_____

DIET JOURNAL

Date: _____

FOOD and BEVERAGE	CALORIE	FIBER	PROTEIN	CARB	FAT
BREAKFAST					
Breakfast Total >					
LUNCH					
Lunch Total >					
DINNER					
Dinner Total >					

SPECIAL DIETARY NOTES:

_____
_____
_____
_____
_____
_____
_____
_____
_____
_____
_____
_____
_____
_____
_____
_____

DIET JOURNAL

Date: _____

FOOD and BEVERAGE	CALORIE	FIBER	PROTEIN	CARB	FAT
BREAKFAST					
Breakfast Total >					
LUNCH					
Lunch Total >					
DINNER					
Dinner Total >					

SPECIAL DIETARY NOTES:

_____
_____
_____
_____
_____
_____
_____
_____
_____
_____
_____
_____
_____
_____
_____

DIET JOURNAL

Date: _____

FOOD and BEVERAGE	CALORIE	FIBER	PROTEIN	CARB	FAT
BREAKFAST					
Breakfast Total >					
LUNCH					
Lunch Total >					
DINNER					
Dinner Total >					

SPECIAL DIETARY NOTES:

_____
_____
_____
_____
_____
_____
_____
_____
_____
_____
_____
_____
_____
_____
_____
_____

DIET JOURNAL

Date: _____

FOOD and BEVERAGE	CALORIE	FIBER	PROTEIN	CARB	FAT
BREAKFAST					
Breakfast Total >					
LUNCH					
Lunch Total >					
DINNER					
Dinner Total >					

SPECIAL DIETARY NOTES:

_____
_____
_____
_____
_____
_____
_____
_____
_____
_____
_____
_____
_____
_____

DIET JOURNAL

Date: _____

FOOD and BEVERAGE	CALORIE	FIBER	PROTEIN	CARB	FAT
BREAKFAST					
Breakfast Total >					
LUNCH					
Lunch Total >					
DINNER					
Dinner Total >					

SPECIAL DIETARY NOTES:

_____
_____
_____
_____
_____
_____
_____
_____
_____
_____
_____
_____
_____
_____
_____

DIET JOURNAL

Date: _____

FOOD and BEVERAGE	CALORIE	FIBER	PROTEIN	CARB	FAT
BREAKFAST					
Breakfast Total >					
LUNCH					
Lunch Total >					
DINNER					
Dinner Total >					

SPECIAL DIETARY NOTES:

_____
_____
_____
_____
_____
_____
_____
_____
_____
_____
_____
_____
_____
_____
_____

DIET JOURNAL

Date: _____

FOOD and BEVERAGE	CALORIE	FIBER	PROTEIN	CARB	FAT
BREAKFAST					
Breakfast Total >					
LUNCH					
Lunch Total >					
DINNER					
Dinner Total >					

SPECIAL DIETARY NOTES:

_____
_____
_____
_____
_____
_____
_____
_____
_____
_____
_____
_____
_____
_____
_____
_____

DIET JOURNAL

Date: _____

FOOD and BEVERAGE	CALORIE	FIBER	PROTEIN	CARB	FAT
BREAKFAST					
Breakfast Total >					
LUNCH					
Lunch Total >					
DINNER					
Dinner Total >					

SPECIAL DIETARY NOTES:

_____
_____
_____
_____
_____
_____
_____
_____
_____
_____
_____
_____
_____
_____

DIET JOURNAL

Date: _____

FOOD and BEVERAGE	CALORIE	FIBER	PROTEIN	CARB	FAT
BREAKFAST					
Breakfast Total >					
LUNCH					
Lunch Total >					
DINNER					
Dinner Total >					

SPECIAL DIETARY NOTES:

_____
_____
_____
_____
_____
_____
_____
_____
_____
_____
_____
_____
_____
_____
_____
_____

DIET JOURNAL

Date: _____

FOOD and BEVERAGE	CALORIE	FIBER	PROTEIN	CARB	FAT
BREAKFAST					
Breakfast Total >					
LUNCH					
Lunch Total >					
DINNER					
Dinner Total >					

SPECIAL DIETARY NOTES:

_____
_____
_____
_____
_____
_____
_____
_____
_____
_____
_____
_____
_____
_____
_____
_____

DIET JOURNAL

Date: _____

FOOD and BEVERAGE	CALORIE	FIBER	PROTEIN	CARB	FAT
BREAKFAST					
Breakfast Total >					
LUNCH					
Lunch Total >					
DINNER					
Dinner Total >					

SPECIAL DIETARY NOTES:

_____
_____
_____
_____
_____
_____
_____
_____
_____
_____
_____
_____
_____
_____
_____
_____

DIET JOURNAL

Date: _____

FOOD and BEVERAGE	CALORIE	FIBER	PROTEIN	CARB	FAT
BREAKFAST					
Breakfast Total >					
LUNCH					
Lunch Total >					
DINNER					
Dinner Total >					

SPECIAL DIETARY NOTES:

_____
_____
_____
_____
_____
_____
_____
_____
_____
_____
_____
_____
_____
_____

DIET JOURNAL

Date: _____

FOOD and BEVERAGE	CALORIE	FIBER	PROTEIN	CARB	FAT
BREAKFAST					
Breakfast Total >					
LUNCH					
Lunch Total >					
DINNER					
Dinner Total >					

SPECIAL DIETARY NOTES:

_____
_____
_____
_____
_____
_____
_____
_____
_____
_____
_____
_____
_____
_____
_____
_____

DIET JOURNAL

Date: _____

FOOD and BEVERAGE	CALORIE	FIBER	PROTEIN	CARB	FAT
BREAKFAST					
Breakfast Total >					
LUNCH					
Lunch Total >					
DINNER					
Dinner Total >					

SPECIAL DIETARY NOTES:

_____
_____
_____
_____
_____
_____
_____
_____
_____
_____
_____
_____
_____
_____
_____
_____

DIET JOURNAL

Date: _____

FOOD and BEVERAGE	CALORIE	FIBER	PROTEIN	CARB	FAT
BREAKFAST					
Breakfast Total >					
LUNCH					
Lunch Total >					
DINNER					
Dinner Total >					

SPECIAL DIETARY NOTES:

DIET JOURNAL

Date: _____

FOOD and BEVERAGE	CALORIE	FIBER	PROTEIN	CARB	FAT
BREAKFAST					
Breakfast Total >					
LUNCH					
Lunch Total >					
DINNER					
Dinner Total >					

SPECIAL DIETARY NOTES:

_____
_____
_____
_____
_____
_____
_____
_____
_____
_____
_____
_____
_____
_____
_____
_____

DIET JOURNAL

Date: _____

FOOD and BEVERAGE	CALORIE	FIBER	PROTEIN	CARB	FAT
BREAKFAST					
Breakfast Total >					
LUNCH					
Lunch Total >					
DINNER					
Dinner Total >					

SPECIAL DIETARY NOTES:

_____
_____
_____
_____
_____
_____
_____
_____
_____
_____
_____
_____
_____
_____

DIET JOURNAL

Date: _____

FOOD and BEVERAGE	CALORIE	FIBER	PROTEIN	CARB	FAT
BREAKFAST					
Breakfast Total >					
LUNCH					
Lunch Total >					
DINNER					
Dinner Total >					

SPECIAL DIETARY NOTES:

_____
_____
_____
_____
_____
_____
_____
_____
_____
_____
_____
_____
_____
_____
_____

DIET JOURNAL

Date: _____

FOOD and BEVERAGE	CALORIE	FIBER	PROTEIN	CARB	FAT
BREAKFAST					
Breakfast Total >					
LUNCH					
Lunch Total >					
DINNER					
Dinner Total >					

SPECIAL DIETARY NOTES:

_____
_____
_____
_____
_____
_____
_____
_____
_____
_____
_____
_____
_____
_____
_____

DIET JOURNAL

Date: _____

FOOD and BEVERAGE	CALORIE	FIBER	PROTEIN	CARB	FAT
BREAKFAST					
Breakfast Total >					
LUNCH					
Lunch Total >					
DINNER					
Dinner Total >					

SPECIAL DIETARY NOTES:
_____
_____
_____
_____
_____
_____
_____
_____
_____
_____
_____
_____
_____
_____
_____

DIET JOURNAL

Date: _____

FOOD and BEVERAGE	CALORIE	FIBER	PROTEIN	CARB	FAT
BREAKFAST					
Breakfast Total >					
LUNCH					
Lunch Total >					
DINNER					
Dinner Total >					

SPECIAL DIETARY NOTES:

_____
_____
_____
_____
_____
_____
_____
_____
_____
_____
_____
_____
_____
_____

DIET JOURNAL

Date: _____

FOOD and BEVERAGE	CALORIE	FIBER	PROTEIN	CARB	FAT
BREAKFAST					
Breakfast Total >					
LUNCH					
Lunch Total >					
DINNER					
Dinner Total >					

SPECIAL DIETARY NOTES:

_____
_____
_____
_____
_____
_____
_____
_____
_____
_____
_____
_____
_____
_____
_____
_____

DIET JOURNAL

Date: _____

FOOD and BEVERAGE	CALORIE	FIBER	PROTEIN	CARB	FAT
BREAKFAST					
Breakfast Total >					
LUNCH					
Lunch Total >					
DINNER					
Dinner Total >					

SPECIAL DIETARY NOTES:

_____
_____
_____
_____
_____
_____
_____
_____
_____
_____
_____
_____
_____
_____
_____
_____

DIET JOURNAL

Date: _____

FOOD and BEVERAGE	CALORIE	FIBER	PROTEIN	CARB	FAT
BREAKFAST					
Breakfast Total >					
LUNCH					
Lunch Total >					
DINNER					
Dinner Total >					

SPECIAL DIETARY NOTES:

_____
_____
_____
_____
_____
_____
_____
_____
_____
_____
_____
_____
_____
_____
_____

DIET JOURNAL

Date: _____

FOOD and BEVERAGE	CALORIE	FIBER	PROTEIN	CARB	FAT
BREAKFAST					
Breakfast Total >					
LUNCH					
Lunch Total >					
DINNER					
Dinner Total >					

SPECIAL DIETARY NOTES:

_____
_____
_____
_____
_____
_____
_____
_____
_____
_____
_____
_____
_____
_____
_____
_____
_____

DIET JOURNAL

Date: _____

FOOD and BEVERAGE	CALORIE	FIBER	PROTEIN	CARB	FAT
BREAKFAST					
Breakfast Total >					
LUNCH					
Lunch Total >					
DINNER					
Dinner Total >					

SPECIAL DIETARY NOTES:

_____
_____
_____
_____
_____
_____
_____
_____
_____
_____
_____
_____
_____
_____
_____
_____

DIET JOURNAL

Date: _____

FOOD and BEVERAGE	CALORIE	FIBER	PROTEIN	CARB	FAT
BREAKFAST					
Breakfast Total >					
LUNCH					
Lunch Total >					
DINNER					
Dinner Total >					

SPECIAL DIETARY NOTES:

_____
_____
_____
_____
_____
_____
_____
_____
_____
_____
_____
_____
_____
_____
_____
_____
_____

DIET JOURNAL

Date: _____

FOOD and BEVERAGE	CALORIE	FIBER	PROTEIN	CARB	FAT
BREAKFAST					
Breakfast Total >					
LUNCH					
Lunch Total >					
DINNER					
Dinner Total >					

SPECIAL DIETARY NOTES:

_____
_____
_____
_____
_____
_____
_____
_____
_____
_____
_____
_____
_____
_____
_____

DIET JOURNAL

Date: _____

FOOD and BEVERAGE	CALORIE	FIBER	PROTEIN	CARB	FAT
BREAKFAST					
Breakfast Total >					
LUNCH					
Lunch Total >					
DINNER					
Dinner Total >					

SPECIAL DIETARY NOTES:

DIET JOURNAL

Date: _____

FOOD and BEVERAGE	CALORIE	FIBER	PROTEIN	CARB	FAT
BREAKFAST					
Breakfast Total >					
LUNCH					
Lunch Total >					
DINNER					
Dinner Total >					

SPECIAL DIETARY NOTES:

_____
_____
_____
_____
_____
_____
_____
_____
_____
_____
_____
_____
_____
_____
_____
_____

DIET JOURNAL

Date: _____

FOOD and BEVERAGE	CALORIE	FIBER	PROTEIN	CARB	FAT
BREAKFAST					
Breakfast Total >					
LUNCH					
Lunch Total >					
DINNER					
Dinner Total >					

SPECIAL DIETARY NOTES:

_____
_____
_____
_____
_____
_____
_____
_____
_____
_____
_____
_____
_____
_____
_____
_____

DIET JOURNAL

Date: _____

FOOD and BEVERAGE	CALORIE	FIBER	PROTEIN	CARB	FAT
BREAKFAST					
Breakfast Total >					
LUNCH					
Lunch Total >					
DINNER					
Dinner Total >					

SPECIAL DIETARY NOTES:

_____
_____
_____
_____
_____
_____
_____
_____
_____
_____
_____
_____
_____
_____
_____
_____
_____

DIET JOURNAL

Date: _____

FOOD and BEVERAGE	CALORIE	FIBER	PROTEIN	CARB	FAT
BREAKFAST					
Breakfast Total >					
LUNCH					
Lunch Total >					
DINNER					
Dinner Total >					

SPECIAL DIETARY NOTES:

_____
_____
_____
_____
_____
_____
_____
_____
_____
_____
_____
_____
_____
_____
_____

DIET JOURNAL

Date: _____

FOOD and BEVERAGE	CALORIE	FIBER	PROTEIN	CARB	FAT
BREAKFAST					
Breakfast Total >					
LUNCH					
Lunch Total >					
DINNER					
Dinner Total >					

SPECIAL DIETARY NOTES:

_____
_____
_____
_____
_____
_____
_____
_____
_____
_____
_____
_____
_____
_____
_____
_____
_____

DIET JOURNAL

Date: _____

FOOD and BEVERAGE	CALORIE	FIBER	PROTEIN	CARB	FAT
BREAKFAST					
Breakfast Total >					
LUNCH					
Lunch Total >					
DINNER					
Dinner Total >					

SPECIAL DIETARY NOTES:

_____
_____
_____
_____
_____
_____
_____
_____
_____
_____
_____
_____
_____
_____
_____

DIET JOURNAL

Date: _____

FOOD and BEVERAGE	CALORIE	FIBER	PROTEIN	CARB	FAT
BREAKFAST					
Breakfast Total >					
LUNCH					
Lunch Total >					
DINNER					
Dinner Total >					

SPECIAL DIETARY NOTES:

_____
_____
_____
_____
_____
_____
_____
_____
_____
_____
_____
_____
_____
_____
_____
_____

DIET JOURNAL

Date: _____

FOOD and BEVERAGE	CALORIE	FIBER	PROTEIN	CARB	FAT
BREAKFAST					
Breakfast Total >					
LUNCH					
Lunch Total >					
DINNER					
Dinner Total >					

SPECIAL DIETARY NOTES:

_____
_____
_____
_____
_____
_____
_____
_____
_____
_____
_____
_____
_____
_____
_____
_____
_____

DIET JOURNAL

Date: _____

FOOD and BEVERAGE	CALORIE	FIBER	PROTEIN	CARB	FAT
BREAKFAST					
Breakfast Total >					
LUNCH					
Lunch Total >					
DINNER					
Dinner Total >					

SPECIAL DIETARY NOTES:

_____
_____
_____
_____
_____
_____
_____
_____
_____
_____
_____
_____
_____
_____
_____

9 781681 851723